Anti-Inflammatory Diet

Guide for enhancing your immune system and stopping inflammation

By

Philip J. Smith

© Copyright 2016 by Philip J. Smith - All rights reserved.

This document is geared towards providing exact and reliable information in regards to the topic and issue covered. The publication is sold on the idea that the publisher is not required to render an accounting, officially permitted, or otherwise, qualified services. If advice is necessary, legal or professional, a practiced individual in the profession should be ordered.

- From a Declaration of Principles which was accepted and approved equally by a Committee of the American Bar Association and a Committee of Publishers and Associations.

In no way is it legal to reproduce, duplicate, or transmit any part of this document by either electronic means or in printed format. Recording of this publication is strictly prohibited, and any storage of this document is not allowed unless with written permission from the publisher. All rights reserved.

The information provided herein is stated to be truthful and consistent, in that any liability, in terms of inattention or otherwise, by any usage or abuse of any policies, processes, or directions contained within is the solitary and utter responsibility of the recipient reader. Under no circumstances will any legal responsibility or blame be held against the publisher for any reparation, damages, or monetary loss due to the information herein, either directly or indirectly.

Respective authors own all copyrights not held by the publisher.

The information herein is offered for informational purposes solely and is universal as so. The presentation of the information is without a contract or any type of guarantee assurance.

The trademarks that are used are without any consent, and the publication of the trademark is without permission or backing by the trademark owner. All trademarks and brands within this book are for clarifying purposes only and are owned by the owners themselves, not affiliated with this document.

Table of Contents

Introduction 1

What are the components of the immune system? 2

How do the defense mechanisms of the immune system act? . 3

First signs that our immune system is endangered 5

Inflammations cure or disease 6

What to eat 9

Which vitamins have the greatest anti-inflammatory potential 13

Exercise as weapon against inflammation 19

How to recognize and prevent harmful inflammatory process in the body 22

Food that can cause inflammation in our body 25

Meal plans 32

    Breakfast recipe No.1 – Toasted rye bread, scrambled eggs, and sesame seeds & yogurt 33

    Snack recipe No.1- Almond cupcakes 35

    Lunch Recipe No.1 – Spiced salmon in foil and cooked brown rice 38

    Dinner recipes No.1 Baked chickpeas, Salad with grilled zucchini 40

    Breakfast No.2 "Yoga" Breakfast 43

    Snack I No. 2 -Smoothie lemon and raspberries 44

    Lunch No.2 - Chicken & broccoli salad 45

Dinner No. 2 Fake cabbage spaghetti with caramelized onions in tomato sauce 47

Breakfast No.3 Whole meal bread with homemade spread sesame tahini 49

Snack I No.3 Blueberry and banana smoothie 51

Lunch recipes No.3 Stuffed Sour red peppers with walnuts 52

Dinner No.3- Mediterranean style Beef and backed potatoes 55

Breakfast No.4 - Polenta with yogurt 57

Snack I No.4 Lemon and sesame Shake 59

Lunch No.4 - Easy turkey salad 60

Dinner No.4:   Minestrone soup, Seafood with asparagus, brown rice, sour red beet salad 62

Breakfast No.5 - Muesli with blueberries and almond milk 65

Snack I No.5 Fruit shake bomb 67

Lunch No.5 Veggie broccoli and oat flakes hamburger 68

Dinner No.5 - Grilled garlic lamb chops with rosemary 71

Breakfast No. 6 – Cinnamon pumpkin waffles 74

Snack I No. 6 – Spicy blueberry sesame smoothie 76

Lunch No. 6: Halibut salad 78

Dinner No.6: Risotto with shiitake mushrooms and vitamin salad 80

Breakfast No.7: Oats muffins with berries 82

Snack I No.7: Ginger banana smoothie 84

Lunch No.7: White Beans baked in the oven, cabbage salad, rye bread 85

Dinner No.7: Avocado & tuna salad 87

Conclusion 93

Introduction

Ask yourself: how many times did you wake up and feel like a train ran over you? If this happens to you, and you didn't consume alcohol beverages the previous night, then probably some inflammatory process has started in your body, because of yours weakened the immune system. Here you will find everything you need to know about inflammatory and how it's linked to your immune system and how can you raise your own awareness of what every human can do to strengthen his/hers defense mechanism and raise function of immune system.

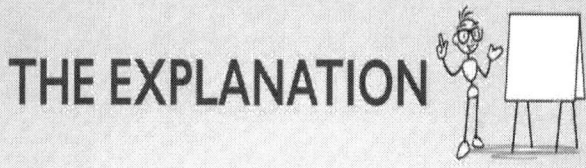

- Physical activity may help flush bacteria out of the lungs and airways. This may reduce your chance of getting a cold, flu, or other airborne illness.

- Exercise causes changes in antibodies and white blood cells (the body's immune system cells that fight disease). These antibodies or white blood cells circulate more rapidly, so they could detect illnesses earlier than they might have before. However, no one knows whether these changes help prevent infections.

- The brief rise in body temperature during and right after exercise may prevent bacteria from growing. This temperature rise may help the body fight infection more effectively. (This is similar to what happens when you have a fever.)

- Exercise slows down the release of stress-related hormones. Some stress increases the chance of illness. Lower stress hormones may protect against illness.

What are the components of the immune system?

Main components of the immune system are Antibodies and bone marrow, spleen and endocrine gland.

Antibodies (also known as immunoglobulins and gamma globulin) are proteins in Y-shaped that respond to specific bacteria, viruses or toxins, called antigens. They are produced by white blood cells.

Antibodies can bind to toxins, disabling their chemical actions or signal that an "attacker "needs to be removed. They are divided into five categories. Their names are generally abbreviated. For example, Immunoglobulin A is abbreviated IgA. Here are all of the abbreviations: IgA, IgD, IgE, IgG, and IgM.

The bone marrow produces new red and white blood cells. Red blood cells are fully formed in the bone marrow and then they enter the bloodstream. The production of white blood cells known as leukocytes also starts in the bone marrow, but part of their development finishes in the thymus, lymph gland, nodes, and spleen.

How do the defense mechanisms of the immune system act?

The immune system acts in several ways: by creating a barrier that prevents bacteria and viruses enter your body. Immune system detects and eliminates bacteria and viruses that manage to get into the body before they have a chance to reproduce and proliferate. The most obvious parts of the immune system are easily visible barriers - our skin, eyes, nose and mouth.

Skin is firm and resistant to many kinds of bacteria, and it also secretes antibacterial substance. Tears and mucus contain an enzyme that destroys the cell walls of many bacteria. And saliva has antibacterial properties, and if some microbes pass through saliva, the next level of defense is stomach acid. For most people, viral and bacterial infections are the most common causes of illness. They usually last until the body becomes immune to those particular microbes and recovers up.

Some hormones in the body can suppress the immune system (steroids and corticosteroids - components of adrenaline hormone). On the other hand, thymosin is a hormone that is formed by the thymus, which is a part of an endocrine gland that encourages lymphocyte production (a lymphocyte is a form of white blood cell). It is believed that production of this hormone can be disturbed if you are constantly under the impact of chronic stress.

You need to know that all tissues of the body are continually bathed in the lymph, a transparent fluid similar to the water, that comes from blood (blood and lymph are body fluids). The lymph system detects and removes bacteria and waste products. The lymph fluid eventually arrives at the lymph nodes, the body 'factories for processing waste material ", which is further processed. Lymph nodes are basically filters that trap germs and other foreign bodies.

The spleen filters the blood looking for foreign cells and old red blood cells that need to be replaced. So, it's very important for you to be aware that with the right kind of food, you can encourage the right parts of your immune system to work properly.

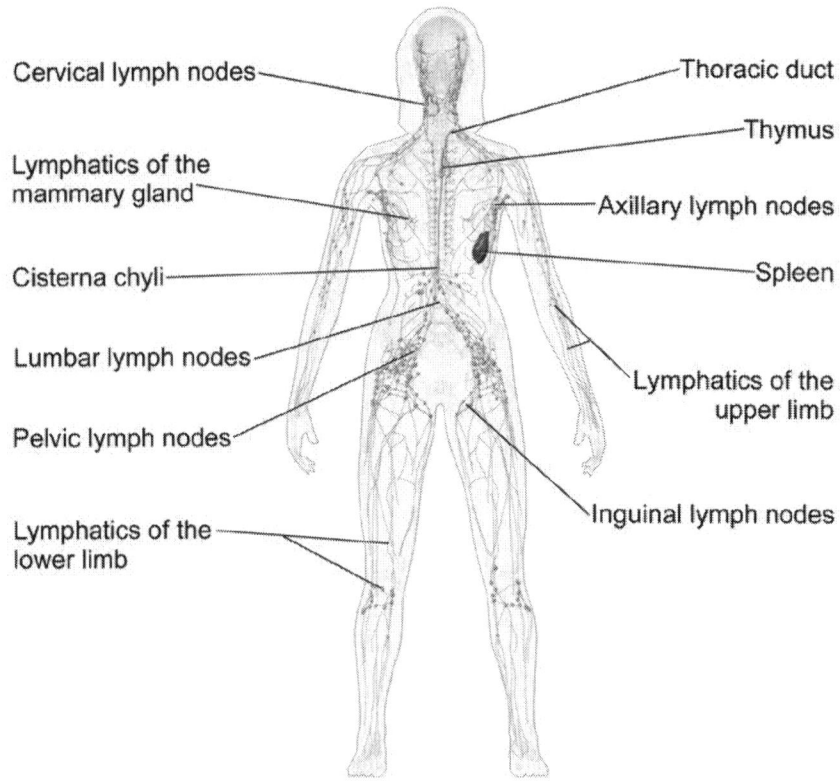

First signs that our immune system is endangered

When we talk about immune system and how can we strengthen it, we need to know that any inflammation is part of the body's immune response and that our body needs to give a huge effort to protect itself, especially if it comes to damaging cells, irritants, or if any pathogens (harmful bacteria's) "attack" our organism. During the defense from inflammatory chemical "messengers" called cytokines (proteins released by cells with the main function of communication between cells), are released[1]. They affect the local blood vessels (in the area of inflammation) which we can feel like an increased heat that occurs in this specific part of the body or as redness, due to increased blood flow. Any kind of inflammatory was originally described in words such as "heat", "pain", "redness", "swelling", etc. What we now know is that all these signs that belong to the inflammatory processes actually aren't part of them – they are a part of the immune response to trauma.

---

[1] Jun-Ming Zhang, MSc, MD and Jianxiong An, MSc, MD. Cytokines, Inflammation and Pain Int Anesthesiol Clin. 2007 Spring; 45(2): 27–37. http://www.ncbi.nlm.nih.gov/pmc/articles/PMC2785020/

Inflammations cure or disease

Any inflammation presents the beginning of the self -healing process. For example, you cut your fingertip with a knife. The blood will very quickly coagulate in the place of the cut, and the bleeding will stop, but the harmful bacteria will probably enter your body. Our immune system will quickly detect the presence of unwanted bacteria and will respond with sending antibodies as the response of activated defense system. This leads to a process of inflammation (pain, redness) that is aimed at fast delivery of antibodies to the place where the unwanted bacteria were observed to be stopped and killed[1].

After this kind of inflammatory response (which is essential and necessary), the inflammatory process should be localized and calming down in order that attacked organ could recover and heal. So, we could freely say that in some cases inflammation process can act as a cure and that inflammation isn't a disease, but a sign that's something is wrong in our body that can lead to serious health problems and cause illness that can even lead to death. I already told you that you can influence on lowering or raising of any inflammatory process with food.

Omega-6 fatty acids that can be found in many kinds of food especially in vegetable oils, mayonnaise, margarine and processed food present a trigger for inflammatory process and increase inflammation that sometimes helps us defense and sometimes just worsen our health[2]. If you enter a high amount of omega 6 fatty acids during a longer time period, it

---

[2] Foods highest in Total Omega-6 fatty acids http://nutritiondata.self.com/foods-000141000000000000000-w.html

will lead to the appearance of insulin resistance, and all this contributes to the development of atherosclerosis and increases the risk of cardiovascular diseases[3]. Omega-3 fatty acids, on the other hand, initiate a process of reducing inflammation and healing.

New research suggests that with the right kind of food and with some lifestyle changes you can reduce inflammation and other risk factors for developing infection or suffering of some diseases.

Obesity is another big trigger for starting of inflammation process because fat cells produce higher amounts of inflammatory chemicals than other cells. When you gain weight, your body will be under the impact of an additional inflammatory process that will increase a chance of getting the disease, and also, it will speed up your aging process.

The ratio between Omega fatty acids (6 and 3) should be from 1: 1 to 5:1 so that the anti-inflammatory system could be in balance. Instead of such a proportions, today's modern nutrition mainly provides ratio between omega 6 and 3 fatty acids is 20:1 to a shocking 50:1

In other words - with the modern way of nutrition we enter more Omega-6 fatty acids and less Omega 3 fatty acids and for this imbalance between these two fatty acids we can be "thankful" to all food manufacturers and modern food

---

[3] Tortosa-Caparrós E, Navas-Carrillo D, Marín F, Orenes-Piñero E. Anti-inflammatory Effects of Omega 3 and Omega 6 Polyunsaturated Fatty Acids in Cardiovascular Disease and Metabolic Syndrome. Department of Cardiology , Hospital Clínico Universitario Virgen de la Arrixaca,Spain. Crit Rev Food Sci Nutr. 2016 Jan 8:0. http://www.ncbi.nlm.nih.gov/pubmed/26745681

industry. This happens while it's increased intake of processed meat products baked and fried foods in relation to the diet of our ancestors which was more natural. So, instead that inflammation occurs only when it is needed - too many people today are in a state of so-called "chronic inflammation" with next symptoms: pain and stiffness, allergy asthma, skin rashes, eczema, psoriasis and premature aging of the skin... etc. It is, therefore, desirable to turn back and establish the natural balance of omega-3 and omega 6 fatty acids in the diet.

What to eat

Unlike many exhausting reductions diets that are requiring fasting or complete exclusion of some types of food from your menu, anti-inflammatory diet cares about the health of one who adheres to, and also such a diet reduces the risk of various diseases it establishes balance in the body and at the same time it will help you achieve optimal body weight.

The basic of an anti-inflammatory diet is hidden in spiced meals. Ask yourself how many spices you have in your kitchen and how many of them do you really use? The world of spices is fascinating and with them, you are always ready to make a flavorful meal or experiment in the kitchen. When you enter spices, you enter lots of antioxidants, and the good news is that you will at the same time lower the amount of salt. If you have not tried the cumin, the best way to learn its flavor is to sprinkle the potatoes and bake them in the oven. If you like to drink hot chocolate add a bit of anise or cinnamon in hot chocolate because they are fuelled with compounds named antioxidants that bind on harmful compounds that are called free radicals in our body and so act anti-inflammatory. The effective dose is typically 0.5-2 teaspoons of cinnamon or anise per day. Instead of coffee I like to start my day with ginger tea, which is a kind of energy bomb for me, it warms me on the inside, stimulates circulation, and an intense aroma wakes all my receptors.

Peppermint oil can recover your guts and influence on lowering irritable bowel syndrome, or IBS (it's a functional gastrointestinal disorder characterized by abdominal pain)[4].

---

[4] Alexander C Ford, Nicholas J Talley, Brennan M R Spiegel, Amy E Foxx-Orenstein, Lawrence Schiller, Eamonn M M Quigley, Paul Moayyedi, *Effect of fibre, antispasmodics, and*

Turmeric (Curcuma) also acts as a powerful anti-inflammatory, antiviral, antibacterial, and antifungal and it even has some anticancer activity. Therefore, it is considered as an effective therapy and prevention of malignant diseases, diabetes, allergies, arthritis, Alzheimer's disease and other chronic diseases[5]. You can add turmeric spices to every salad dressing it will give an extra nutritional value and orange-yellow shade, or you can use it with any salad with eggs while it will give even stronger yellow color and additional nutritional benefits.

If you like brown rice mix turmeric powder with brown rice, raisins, and cashew nuts. Although turmeric is generally the main ingredient of curry powder, some people like to add a bit of spice when preparing curry. Turmeric or curry powder spices are great for complementing flavors of cooked lentil and cauliflower. Don't forget the basil, parsley while they will improve your immune system because they inhibit the growth of harmful bacteria, yeasts, and molds.

I need to warn you about another **Myth: Citrus Fruits Cause Inflammation**

"Many websites are filled with warnings for people who suffer from arthritis to avoid citrus fruits because they supposedly promote inflammation. On the other side, citrus fruits are rich in vitamin C, and the long-term Framingham Heart Study in Massachusetts showed OA progression dropped by more than half people who consumed at least 152 milligrams of vitamin C

---

peppermint oil in the treatment of irritable bowel syndrome: systematic review and meta-analysisBMJ 2008;337:a2313 http://www.bmj.com/content/337/bmj.a2313

[5] Thorne Research, Inc. jjurenka@thorne.com. Anti-inflammatory properties of curcumin, a major constituent of Curcuma longa: a review of preclinical and clinical research. Altern Med Rev. 2009 Jun;14(2):141-53. http://www.ncbi.nlm.nih.gov/pubmed/19594223

a day. Bottom Line: Don't shy away from citrus fruits. Their vitamin C might protect against OA pain and is critical in the formation of the major components of cartilage. In addition, vitamin C is an antioxidant that can quench cartilage-damaging free radicals".[6]

If you follow the following dietary rules, you can reduce inflammation in your body.

- Eat lots of fresh fruits and vegetables, if possible, organic. Give preferences to fruit rich in antioxidants (all kind of berries and black grapes) and veggies from the cabbage family and dark green leafy veggies (spinach, chard).

- Use fatty fish in your diet more often (2 -3 times a week), because it is an excellent source of omega-3 unsaturated fats and it has the right or natural ratio between omega 3 and 6 fatty acids, or you can drink a teaspoon of fish oil a day during the winter season.

- All food that you cook sautés or bake on natural oils such as lard, tallow or olive oil.

- Instead of eating refined grains use integral grains because they don't contain added sugar, and they belong to food with low glycemic index (such as oats and barley).

- Choose meat that has not been treated with hormones. From cheeses select fresh goat cheese.

---

[6] Arthritis Food Myths Arthritis Foundation National Office http://www.arthritis.org/living-with-arthritis/arthritis-diet/anti-inflammatory/food-myths-arthritis.php

- During the day, drink plenty of water, and it would be wise to drink mint tea (it contains peppermint) or green tea after each main meal because it will help your body cleanse the liver and pancreas.

- As antioxidants are preferred in anti- inflammatory diet you can on a daily base drink one glass of red wine or eat a smaller piece of dark chocolate (70-72% of cocoa contents).

As I previously said, spices have powerful anti-inflammatory effects like oregano ginger, turmeric, and chili peppers, so it is good to eat them in smaller amounts as often as possible (never overdo it with any kind of herbs (spices), because they contain a lot of antioxidants and in higher amounts they will act toxic or even develop lack of minerals like iron, zinc and calcium[7]).Do not use antioxidant supplements to replace a healthy diet, eat real food, and very soon you will see all the benefits from it.

---

[7] Antioxidants American dietetic association http://www.womenfirst.net/pdf/ADA/ADA_Antioxidants.pdf

Which vitamins have the greatest anti-inflammatory potential

Vitamin A is one of the strongest natural antioxidants, which means that one of its many abilities is to protect our body from various harmful free radicals that are created as a by-product of metabolism. Lack of vitamin A is rare nowadays except in developed countries in Africa and Asia. Vitamin A deficiency is most associated with inflammation of the intestines, lungs, and skin. In nature it can be found in two forms as "retinoid" it's tied to the food of animal origin and in a form of pigments known as "carotenoids" it is a part of plant food.

A retinoid form of vitamin A is above all important when it comes to night vision, for proper pregnancy and childhood growth. It participates in the creation of red blood cells and acts in a form of strong immune response when it comes to resistance to infectious diseases because it enhances the activity of white blood cells.

Food richest with vitamin A in a form of retinoid:

- shrimps
- eggs
- cow milk
- cheddar cheese made from whole milk
- yogurt
- salmon

When it comes to carotenoids form, the primary function of vitamin A is to act as an antioxidant and anti-inflammatory nutrient. Carotenoids are more present in plant food with very vibrant colors like orange and dark green.

Food richest with vitamin A in a form of carotenoids is:

- carrots
- sweet potato
- Spinach
- kale
- swiss chard
- greens

So, if you eat greens and eggs at least twice a week, you don't need to worry about vitamin A deficiency. The recommended daily amount of vitamin A for adult men is 900 mcg and 700 mcg for adult women.

Another vitamin that is linked with numerous inflammatory diseases including appearing signs of rheumatism, arthritis, lupus or type I diabetes is vitamin D. We all know that vitamin D is essential for helping calcium to be effectively absorbed in our skeleton (build and maintain healthy bones). So, even if you intake enough calcium, but in the same time, not enough vitamin D, it will result with osteomalacia at adults (softening of the bones), that causes bone pain and muscle weakness. The good news is that just by simply exposing your unclothed skin to sunlight your body will start to produce Vitamin D after 3 - 4 days of exposure to the sun rays. Nevertheless, any excessive exposure to the sun can potentially lead to skin cancer under the influence of dangerous UV sun rays. The Skin Cancer Foundation recommends that we can get our optional daily intake of vitamin D from food sources like:

- Fatty fish as tuna, salmon, sardines, herring, mackerel
- 2 a week of fish oil,
- 2 – 3 during a week of egg yolks,
- Beef liver
- A cup of Fortified milk every second day

Vitamin E is another key antioxidant with anti-inflammatory properties because our body needs this vitamin to keep the immune system strong enough to act against harmful impact of various bacteria and viruses. Vitamin E participates in the formation of red blood cells, and all of our cells use vitamin E for normal functioning. The easiest way to make sure you are getting enough vitamin E is by including seeds as snacks or as part of a meal such as a pumpkin, sunflowers, chia, sesame or flax seeds. You only need 15 mg of vitamin E and the best food to achieve this amount is to combine some of the next ingredients:

- A handful of Seeds
- One Avocado
- 2 tbsp. of Olive oil
- 1 – 2 cups of dark green veggies
- Few pieces of nuts

- Fatty fish

All of those above mentioned vitamins belong to fat-soluble vitamins, which means that you need to consume food where those vitamins are a part of nutrients, so they could dissolve in your body.

There is one more group of vitamins known as water-soluble vitamins. Vitamins from B group and vitamin C belong to this group.

All B vitamins assist in the conversion of food into "fuel" needed for creating energy for our body. Unfortunately, our body can't store any reserve when water soluble vitamins are in matter, so you need to consume food with water soluble vitamins on a daily base, unlike vitamins that are soluble in fats because our body can make reserves of it.

You also need to be aware that using some medications mixed with chronic inflammation can also cause lower levels of vitamin B6 for example. Vitamin B6 deficiency leads to increased risk of inflammation-related diseases as atherosclerosis or rheumatoid arthritis.

Food high in vitamin B6:

- Whole grain flour
- Bananas
- Poultry meat
- Fatty fish
- Milk

- Cheese
- Lentils
- Brown rice

Remember that low intake of vitamin B6 causes inflammation which then leads to many serious diseases[8].

Vitamin C is probably the most known antioxidant, and we all know that it protects our body from the flu. But its role in the body is manifold, such as: helping the creation of collagen (builder element of skin) and it provides structure for our tendons and muscles, vascular tissues, and bones. Whenever we have some visible wound, vitamin C helps our body to heal it faster. Smokers have lower levels of vitamin C than nonsmokers in the blood, and it will affect the speed of blood flow in the bloodstream.

If you now think that you will solve some inflammatory process easier if you use some supplements instead of real food that contains those vitamins, you are pretty wrong. It's true that in some cases supplements can help us and positively impact on our body, but don't ever keep from your mind that they are just supplements and that they are made in laboratories. By using just common sense, which one would you rather use: something natural through food or something made in a lab? I prefer real one from organic food.

Vitamins I mentioned above are the ones that have the most influence on the appearance of inflammation when there are not enough of them in our body, but of course, they are not the

---

[8] Lotto V, Choi SW, Friso S. Department of Medicine, University of Verona School of Medicine, Policlinico GB Rossi, Verona, Italy. Vitamin B6: a challenging link between nutrition and inflammation in CVD. Br J Nutr. 2011 Jul;106(2):183-95 http://www.ncbi.nlm.nih.gov/pubmed/21486513

only vitamins our body needs. Our body is a complex machine that needs a lot of elements, not just vitamins, to function properly.

When we are talking about combating against inflammation, then we need to include some kind of exercise too.

Exercise as weapon against inflammation

I need to admit that in one part of my life I became pretty lazy when it comes to exercising, especially when I started to drive my car, so almost everything was within my reach. I forgot how physical activity improves everything - from mood to physical appearance. Exercise will help you in the prevention of overweight or with maintaining body weight after a diet or a big weight loss.

When you do physical activity, you burn calories. The more intense activity gets you burn more calories. You do not need to devote much of your free time for exercise to benefit in terms of body weight or a healthier lifestyle.

It's very interesting to know that exercise influences on inflammation process in our body a lot. In the same time, it can reduce inflammation, but also increase it. I already wrote in previous chapters about how inflammation can at the same time be a cure or a first sign that something serious is happening in our body. So, depending on the context, increased inflammation is either a good thing or a bad thing. There are many types of research that confirmed reduced inflammatory markers in our body after regular long-term exercise. In one of those studies, 82 participants who suffer from diabetes type2 were included and tracked for over a year[9]. They performed exercise based on low-intensity physical activity, and the results were amazing. Not only that

---

[9] Balducci S, Zanuso S, Nicolucci A, Fernando F, Cavallo S, Cardelli P, Fallucca S, Alessi E, Letizia C, Jimenez A, Fallucca F, Pugliese G. Anti-inflammatory effect of exercise training in subjects with type 2 diabetes and the metabolic syndrome is dependent on exercise modalities and independent of weight loss. Metabolic Fitness Association, Monterotondo, Rome, Italy. Nutr Metab Cardiovasc Dis. 2010 Oct;20(8):608-17. http://www.ncbi.nlm.nih.gov/pubmed/19695853

they lowered inflammation process in the body, but they also have brought the insulin levels which were released into the bloodstream under control. Therefore, we could freely say that any kind of moderate exercise will have an anti-inflammatory effect and healing effect too.

You have probably felt unpleasant pain in the muscles after a hard workout, training or another form of physical activity that you have not practiced for a long time (skiing, swimming even longer running), which made very difficult for you to move around. Don't worry; you aren't sick, and those symptoms present a signal from your body when you are under inflammation process.

Muscle inflammation appears due to micro - pitting of muscle fiber that, "tears" your muscle tissue and lactic acid appear in the "cracks" of muscle tissue, and lactic acid is the main culprit of muscle inflammation after exercise. One of the well-known methods for the treatment of muscle inflammation is preparations based on acetylsalicylic acid like ordinary aspirin that will neutralize the impact of lactic acid.

Now, you are probably scratching your head and asking yourself – why the heck would I deliberately provoke muscle inflammation and hurt my muscles? Well, to keep them in a good shape, because our muscles allow all movements of the body, from the blink of an eye, or a jump. Even, digestion and blood flow throughout the body depends on muscles, so you need to develop your muscles constantly.

Muscles are largely composed of proteins, and when it comes to disruption of muscles (when there is inflammation happening), muscle cells use lactic acid as a source of energy, and that leads to muscle growth. Muscle tissue can't growth, and new synthesis of muscle cell can't appear if proteins that muscle made previously aren't broken down.

Except better physical look, you will tighten up muscles and protect your bones too. So, the least you can do for yourself is to involve any kind of exercise for at least half an hour in your daily schedule. Don't tell me that you don't have time for a quick walk or to go the gym.

How to recognize and prevent harmful inflammatory process in the body

Fighting inflammation is not a naive thing at all. Today, due to the high desire to live longer and without pain, many pharmaceutical companies are investing huge efforts in order to offer effective medicines for controlling and winning inflammatory processes in the body. Is this indeed what we need?

Millions of people worldwide suffer from some sort of rheumatic diseases. Rheumatic diseases are a set of various diseases with common symptoms like inflammation, swelling and pain in the joints, muscles, tendons and reduced mobility. Unlike muscle inflammation that occurs immediately after strenuous physical exercise, harmful inflammations are associated with pain that lasts longer than a month, and that usually occurs shortly after waking up. So, if you find yourself here, then you should go to the nearest rheumatologist as soon as possible because this is a reliable sign of the appearance of some form of the rheumatoid disease.

Unfortunately, most forms of rheumatic diseases belong to the so-called autoimmune diseases that occur when the immune system, which normally should defend the body from harmful environmental influences, begins to attack its own cells. It is believed that the cause of these kinds of diseases lies in the combination of genetic and modern lifestyle.

When we talk about genetic factors, you can do almost nothing, but when the way of our lifestyle is in the matter, we can take much more, like changing our bad habits and addictions. By that, I don't only think about how to resolve an alcohol or smoking addiction. I mentioned the most common bad addictions that will probably extend any inflammatory process that began in your body. Among bad habits, except poor or wrong kind of diet, a lack of physical exercise is crucial for bringing your body under the chronical influence of inflammation, which then leads to a development of many serious kinds of illnesses. I emphasize this, just to let you know that sometimes you can't blame your forefathers, destiny or God, for some heavy physical condition that befalls you. The only person you can blame is yourself.

Even so, that some inflammatory rheumatic diseases can't be prevented with early diagnosis and early treatment you can favorably influence on their flow. It seems that the modern way of life, with nutrition that is full of added sugars and saturated fat, enriched with many kinds of flavors and additives, and with little or no physical activity, makes much easier to any inflammatory processes to start in our body.

One of the common signs that your body lost the battle with inflammation and that your immune system failed can be:

- ➢ Obesity as No.1 presents one of the first signs that we are under inflammatory process. Over 300 million people suffer from obesity.10 Reducing body weight will stimulate fat cells to produce fewer cytokines ("messengers" for beginning of inflammation).

- ➢ Gingivitis is a problem that occurs in almost 80% of the adult population. Gingivitis refers to the inflammatory

---

[10] Controlling the global obesity epidemic World Health Organization http://www.who.int/nutrition/topics/obesity/en/

processes that arise in the tissues immediate lined to the teeth as a reaction to bacterial accumulations (dental plaque) on the teeth[11]. Just wash your teeth properly and you will probably avoid this inflammatory process.

> ➢ High blood pressure or constantly feeling tired are also one of the first signs that some inflammatory process started in your body, so in such cases, it would be wise to visit a doctor as soon as possible.

The good thing is that there are many ways you can fight inflammation problems: get enough sleep, smoking cessation, regular exercise, and adequate nutrition.

---

[11] Walter J. Loesche and Natalie S. Grossman Periodontal Disease as a Specific, albeit Chronic, Infection: Diagnosis and Treatment School of Dentistry and Department of Microbiology and Immunology, School of Medicine, University of Michigan, American Society for Microbiology Clin Microbiol Rev. 2001 Oct; 14(4): 727–752. http://www.ncbi.nlm.nih.gov/pmc/articles/PMC89001/

Food that can cause inflammation in our body

In the order to prevent inflammation in the body I strongly recommend you to avoid food that can potentially be a trigger for inflammation such as:

✓ **Sugar and processed starches.**

Excessive use of highly processed carbohydrates (sugar, white flour and all products made from them) is one of the main culprits. Every time when you eat some "empty "carbohydrates (pure sugar), without dietary fibers, it will result in rising of your blood sugar levels in the body.

This then leads to greater production of insulin, to overthrow blood sugar from blood back to the previous state by causing the immune response to inflammatory process. And it happens every time you eat food with added white sugar (sucrose) and high fructose corn syrup because of its high content in processed and artificial food products.

Consumption of artificially derived fructose can lead to a state of chronic inflammation associated with obesity, insulin resistance, diabetes, fatty liver disease, chronic renal diseases, and cancers. Those kinds of sugars are commonly found in soft drinks, sweetener packets, ready to eat cereals, snack foods, some dairy products like fruit yogurt, but also in some medications than can be more harmful if you aren't aware that you have in taken them and so unwillingly caused some inflammation process.

Unlike glucose when we enter fructose, it can't be used as an energy source by our cells straight away; it needs to be converted in the liver, intestine and kidney into glucose, lactate or fatty acids first and only after that can be used as an energy source[12]. Lots of studies showed that nutrition that is based on everyday consumption of high-fructose corn syrup sweetened (HFCS), may be associated with increased risk of developing rheumatoid arthritis; women are more susceptible to become ill compared to men[13].

So, next time you go to a restaurant thinks twice before you order you drink. The food industry uses corn derivatives in huge quantities in their products. They also use corn syrup fructose, corn oil and corn starch that are cheap and easily available. In this form, processed corn raises the level of sugar in the blood, which leads to increased production of insulin which in turn causes an inflammatory reaction.

✓ **Industry Vegetable Oils**

Many vegetable oils are rich in omega-6 fats, which disturbs the balance of essential omega-3 and omega-6 fats in the body. Although omega-6 fatty acids are not harmful themselves, when this balance is disrupted, it will cause inflammation as I mentioned in previous chapters. I need to especially warn you about fake olive oil that can be found on the market worldwide. It looks like real olive oil and it even smells the same, but it is fake. Instead of olive, many manufacturers make this oil from soya beans seeds with some artificial flavor and green audible color.

---

[12] Campos VC, Tappy L. Physiological handling of dietary fructose-containing sugars: implications for health.Faculty of Biology and Medicine, Department of Physiology, Lausanne University School of Biology and Medicine, Lausanne, Switzerland. <u>Int J Obes (Lond).</u> 2016 Mar;40 Suppl 1:S6-S11 http://www.ncbi.nlm.nih.gov/pubmed/27001645

[13] DeChristopher LR, Uribarri J, Tucker KL. Intake of high-fructose corn syrup sweetened soft drinks, fruit drinks and apple juice is associated with prevalent arthritis in US adults, aged 20-30 years. Molecular Biology, NY Medical College, Valhalla, NY, USA. <u>Nutr Diabetes.</u> 2016 Mar 7;6:e199 http://www.ncbi.nlm.nih.gov/pubmed/26950480

Even the European Commission for the Environment, Public Health, and Food Safety has warned that olive oil is one of the products that is most often falsified[14].

Top 10 products that are most at risk of food fraud	
1.	Olive oil
2.	Fish
3.	Organic foods
4.	Milk
5.	Grains
6.	Honey and maple syrup
7.	Coffee and tea
8.	Spices (such as saffron and chili powder)
9.	Wine
10.	Certain fruit juices

Table 1. Is based on Development and Application of a Database of Food Ingredient Fraud and Economically Motivated Adulteration from 1980 to 2010 / Moore, J, Spink, J, and Lipkus, M. In Journal of Food Science, 2012, Volume 77 (Number 4), p. R118-R126

---

[14] European Commission for the Environment, Public Health and Food Safety REPORT on the food crisis, fraud in the food chain and the control there of (2013/2091(INI)) from 4 December 2013 Document selected : A7-0434/2013 http://www.europarl.europa.eu/sides/getDoc.do?pubRef=-//EP//TEXT+REPORT+A7-2013-0434+0+DOC+XML+V0//EN

Olive oil is relatively easy to falsify with other kinds of oil. If manufacturers add just 10ml on a whole bottle of considerably cheaper oil, then the fake olive oil will retain its clarity. Falsely oil can be detected only by analysis of fatty acid composition because any edible oil has a different composition of fatty acids. The most common plagiarism of oil variants is to replace it with beets or soy oil, and the color can be adjusted by adding chlorophyll and beta-carotene. Therefore, if you are able to purchase your goods from reliable food manufacturer even if you pay a bit more for them, buy it because you can only then be sure that you have bought the real thing.

How to recognize real olive oil?

There are a lot of advice on how to choose and recognize the right olive oil, but this way is often mentioned. To determine whether you bought the original or plagiarism; put oil in the fridge for more than ten hours. If it thickens and hardens, then it is real olive oil, and if not there are supplements, and it is fake. It is best if you leave it in the fridge for 24 hours because this test has its flaws.

Olives are different, and the time of reading can influence on how much oil is needed to solidify. Olive oil is 70 percent monounsaturated, and sunflower oil is 70 percent polyunsaturated. When you keep oil in a cold place for some time (ex: in the freezer), monounsaturated fats become solid or semi-solid and polyunsaturated stay as they were, liquid.

So, olive oil will thicken and harden, and sunflower won't. Extra virgin olive oil should solidify in the fridge (of course, not like fat or butter). Do not keep it in the fridge and be sure to buy it in dark bottles (it is important that you keep it away from the light). The misconception is that it is not good to fry olive oil.

Experts note that it is even better to fry on olive than on sunflower oil because it has better quality and it is more stable. But the problem is, of course, the price because olive oil is a lot more expensive.

✓ **Food rich in artificial trans fats**

There are two types of trans fats: ones that can be found in natural form and the ones that are produced in labs. The natural trans fats are produced mainly in guts of some animals like cows, sheep's or goats for example and those trans fats then become a natural part of milk, dairy products, meat and meat products.

Our body can "recognize" these fats, so they don't have a harmful impact on our body, unlike artificial trans fats that "attack" our blood vessels and clog them, because they can't be metabolized by our body, so they stick to blood vessels inner walls.

Artificial trans fats are unfortunately still a part of many food products such as ready to eat meals (frozen or fresh) many bakery products like donuts, cakes, cookies, biscuits, pie crusts, crackers, and stick margarine, because they are made with cheaper kinds of ingredient to help prolonged their shelf life.

Even if it says "0 grams of trans fats" on a label of some product it doesn't mean that such product doesn't contain any artificial trans fats amount, but it means that trans fats per serving are equal, or a bit lower than 0.5 grams and food manufacturers in such cases can freely put that their product doesn't contain any artificial trans fats.

Even the US Food and Drug Administration (FDA) made a preliminary determination , not so long ago (in November of 2013), that moderately hydrogenated oils are no longer generally recognized as safe (GRAS) for human food[15].

When we enter artificial trans fats (hydrogenated oils that are found in many processed products like margarine), then more of bad cholesterol know as LDL will be created, which then again promotes inflammation.

✓ **Food that contains many artificial chemicals**

Have you ever tried to read any list of food additives on the label of some food product out loud? For me it was hard just to spell it, I didn't even try to read some of them. I am not a chemist, but I suppose that even for them some of those additives are hard to write. The human body was not made to digest artificial components such as additives, preservatives, artificial colors and other artificial substances that can be found in the processed products. Since the body does not recognize them as food, it's logical that some inflammatory reaction starts in the organism.

Some of them will "kill" our feeling of satiety and even when we aren't hungry you will continue to eat because some additives impact on our brain function and prevent it from sending a signal to our stomach that it's full[16].

---

[15] US Food and Drug Administration "Protecting and Promoting Your Health." http://www.fda.gov/Food/PopularTopics/ucm373922.htm

[16] He K, Du S, Xun P, Sharma S, Wang H, Zhai F, Popkin B, "Consumption of monosodium glutamate in relation to incidence of overweight

Unfortunately, we can't avoid many of them because they are present almost everywhere, from juices, dry mixes for beverages and desserts, up to sausages and even in chewing gum. So, to avoid them, prepare your own meals and try to avoid edible colors when you prepare some cake as much as you can, instead of them use real fruits or homemade syrups.

Give priority to steaks instead of sausages, drink water instead of artificial juices or make your own juice without added colors or sweeteners.

---

in Chinese adults," China Health and Nutrition Survey (CHNS). Departments of Nutrition and Epidemiology, Gillings School of Global
Public Health, University of North Carolina. *Am J Clin Nutr.* 98, no. 6 (2011 Jun): 1328–36. http://ajcn.nutrition.org/content/94/3/958.2.full

Meal plans

When you are making your weekly meal plan, it would be good to firstly choose what will you and your family eats during that week. My advice is that you, first of all, make your grocery list and stick to it when you go shopping so you will not only buy healthier food but at the same time you will save money and above all think about your health. Because I take care of what kind of food me and my family use I decided to engage a professional dietitian nutritionist who provided me with a 7-day meal plan with all recipes which will I now share with you so you can stick to it for a whole month. This meal plan will show you a pattern on how to eat healthier and what groceries you need to choose to reduce the inflammation process in your body. This way you will easily learn how to choose ingredients for your meals.

Breakfast recipe No.1 – Toasted rye bread, scrambled eggs, and sesame seeds & yogurt

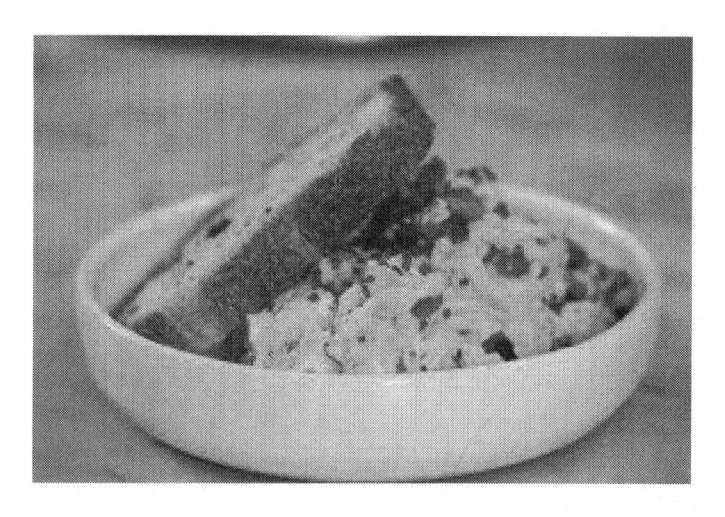

Preparation Time for <u>scrambled eggs:</u> 2 minutes.

Cooking time: 3 minutes

Number of serves: 1

<u>Ingredients:</u>

- 2 large eggs
- 1 tsp. of olive oil
- 1 tbsp. of fresh dill
- 1 tbsp. of fresh parsley
- 1 tbsp. of sesame seeds
- 1 slice of toast rye bread

- 1 cup of yogurt

Preparation:

1. Whisk up the eggs in a medium mixing bowl and add sesame seeds.

2. Cook eggs with sesame seeds on medium heat in a small frying pan, let it brown on one side for a minute; then flip and serve.

3. Combine eggs with fresh parsley and dill, before cooking them or when you serve them on the plate just sprinkle parsley over it. Serve with toast and yogurt.

Nutritional information: This combination of food is very high in calcium, phosphorus, and vitamin B12. Phosphorus is needed for the growth, protection, and repair of all tissues and cells, and it also helps reduce muscle pain after exercising. This combination provides not just enough energy for the beginning of a day but also impacts on the regulation of your guts[17].

---

[17] Imanishi Y, Koyama H, Inaba M, Okuno S, Nishizawa Y, Morii H, Otani S. Phosphorus intake regulates intestinal function and polyamine metabolism in uremia. Department of Biochemistry, Osaka City University Medical School, Japan. <u>Kidney Int.</u> 1996 Feb;49(2):499-505. http://www.ncbi.nlm.nih.gov/pubmed/8821836

Snack recipe No.1- Almond cupcakes

Preparation time: 60 minutes

Baking time: 20 minutes

Ingredients for 24 medium sized:

- 4 oz (115 g) of unsalted butter
- 3.5 (100 g) of sugar
- 2 tsp of vanilla sugar
- 2 eggs
- 6.7 oz (190 g) of almond flour
- 1 full tsp of baking powder
- 4 oz (120 ml) of nonfat milk

For icing cream:

- 2 cups of heavy cream
- 9 oz (250 g) of dark chocolate (70% cocoa)
- 1 tsp. of gelatin (dissolved according to manufacturer's instructions)'

For decoration: a handful of coarsely chopped almonds

Preparation:

1. Preheat the oven to 356°F or 180°C.

2. Arrange cupcake papers in a baking pan for muffins and set aside.

3. Whip the sugar, vanilla sugar, and butter creamy mass with a mixer on high speed for a couple of minutes or until it is well blended.

4. Separate the egg yolks from the egg whites into two mixing bowls and whisk egg whites with a mixer until it becomes sturdy (3-5 minutes). Set aside.

5. Add separated eggs yolks in a mixing bowl with butter and mix it thoroughly until all ingredients are well combined.

6. Stir in mixed almond flour with baking powder, add milk and mix until you get a smooth mixture.

7. With a wooden spoon gently stir whisked eggs whites to unite the batter (it will become fluffy).

8. Pour batter into the prepared pan but leave enough space for the growth of cupcakes.

9. Bake for about 20 minutes or you can check if cupcakes are baked by inserting a wooden pick in centers of cupcakes and if it comes out clean, they are baked. Cool in a pan on a wire rack 5 minutes before removing from pan to rack.

10. While the cupcakes are baking, make the cream: warm the cream in a saucepan over medium heat (be careful

not to boil it) and add the broken chocolate and stir until the chocolate is melted.

11. Turn off the stove and when the mass cools, transfer it to a mixing bowl, whisk it and add dissolved gelatin, mix for another minute and leave it for 5 minutes in a fridge. With baker's decorating tool set arrange the icing cream over the cupcakes and sprinkle with some chopped almonds. Keep them in a fridge until serving.

Nutritional information: Almonds are incredibly high with antioxidants[18]. Butter is a rich source of easily absorbed vitamin A, and butter also provides the perfect balance of omega-3 and omega-6 fats, and all of this will keep your endocrine system in top shape and lower any eventual inflammation process. Dairy products consumption isn't associated with inflammatory biomarkers levels and other cardiometabolic risk factors[19].

---

[18] http://superfoodly.com/orac-value/nuts-almonds
[19] Rashidi Pour Fard N, Karimi M, Baghaei MH, Haghighatdoost F, Rouhani MH, Esmaillzadeh A, Azadbakht L. Dairy consumption, cardiovascular risk factors and inflammation in elderly subjects Shahid Motahari Hospital, Fooladshahr, Isfahan, Iran. ARYA Atheroscler. 2015 Nov;11(6):323-31. http://www.ncbi.nlm.nih.gov/pubmed/26862340

Lunch Recipe No.1 – Spiced salmon in foil and cooked brown rice

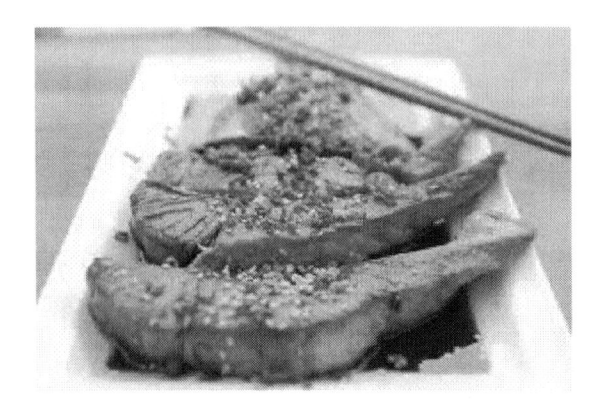

Preparation time: 20 minutes:

Cooking time: 25 minutes

Number of serves: 4

<u>Ingredients for Salmon:</u>

- a small bunch of beet leaves
- ½ a tsp. of sea salt
- 12 mint leaves
- 4 crushed garlic cloves,
- 1 tbsp. of oregano
- 2 red hot chili peppers,
- 5 tbsps. of fresh lime juice
- 2 tbsp. of olive oil

- 4 x 5oz (140g) of salmon fillets

- 4 cups of cooked brown rice as a side dish (1.5 uncooked rice and 4 cups of boiling salted water to cook it in)

Preparation:

1. Preheat the oven to 430°F or 220°C.

2. Blend the beet and mint leaves, salt, garlic, oregano and chilies together in a food processor to make a rough paste. Add the lime juice, olive oil and process until fairly smooth. Spoon the sauce into a bowl and combine with the salmon, then marinate for 20 minutes.

3. Place the marinated fish in the center of the foil, wrap the ends of the foil to form a spiral shape so that it's completely sealed and no steam can escape.

4. Place the foil packet on a heavy large baking sheet. Repeat until all of the salmon has been individually wrapped in foil and placed on the baking sheet. Bake until the salmon is just cooked through, it takes about 25 minutes. Serve with cooked brown rice and some salad (tomatoes, cucumber or mixed salad).

Nutritional information: Salmon has small bioactive protein molecules (called bioactive peptides) that can possibly provide special carry for insulin effectiveness, joint cartilage, and control of inflammation and it has beneficial effects against cardiovascular diseases[20].

---

[20] Arita M, Bianchini F, Aliberti J, Sher A, Chiang N, Hong S, Yang R, Petasis NA, Serhan CN. Stereochemical assignment, antiinflammatory properties, and receptor for the omega-3 lipid mediator resolvin E1. *J Exp Med.* 2005 Mar 7;201(5):713-22. 2005. PMID:15753205. http://www.ncbi.nlm.nih.gov/pubmed/15753205

Dinner recipes No.1 Baked chickpeas, Salad with grilled zucchini

Preparation time: 10 minutes:

Cooking time: 20 – 25 minutes

Number of serves: 6

Ingredients:

- 12 oz (340g) of drained chickpeas
- 2 tbsp. of olive oil
- 1 tbsp. of dried turmeric
- 2 cloves of chopped garlic
- Pinch of black pepper

Preparation:

1. Preheat oven to 380°F or 200°C.
2. Dry chickpeas with a paper towel.
3. Pour the oil and sprinkle with turmeric, pepper and garlic. Place the chickpeas in an ovenproof dish, cover with lid or aluminum foil and bake for 20 to 30 minutes.
4. Serve with grilled zucchini salad.

For Salad with grilled zucchini:

Preparation time: 10 minutes:

Cooking time: 5 minutes

Number of serves: 1

Ingredients:

- 3 medium sized zucchini (cut in strips)
- 2 tbsp. of olive oil
- 2 beetroots (medium size 2" did,)
- 3 medium carrots
- 14 pieces of coarsely chopped almonds
- 4 oz (115 g)of goat cheese
- ½ a hand of raisins
- Pinch of Salt and pepper
- Juice from one freshly squeezed lemon
- 1 ½ tbsp. of cold-pressed olive oil

Preparation:

1. Pour olive oil in a deeper court, about 2 tbsp, heat it on medium high, add striped zucchini and fry over medium heat for about 10 minutes, stirring frequently until the liquid evaporates (about 5 minutes).

2. When done, transfer to a bowl in which you serve the salad. Cut carrots and beets in strips too and mix all others ingredients together. Serve with baked chickpeas.

Nutritional information: Chickpeas contains significant amounts of fiber and mineral selenium, and so it stops inflammation. Choline is another very important nutrient in chickpeas that helps us sustain the structure of cellular membranes; it assists in the transmission of nerve impulses, and it supports the absorption of fats and reduces chronic inflammation[21].

---

[21] Megan Ware RDN LD.Chickpeas: Health Benefits, Nutritional Information MediLexicon International Ltd, Bexhill-on-Sea, UK http://www.medicalnewstoday.com/articles/280244.php

Breakfast No.2 "Yoga" Breakfast

Preparation time: 5 minutes:

Cooking time: - minutes

Number of serves: 1

Ingredients:

- 3 Tbsp of minced barley,
- 2 pieces of dried apricots,
- 4 pieces of coarsely chopped walnuts
- 3 prunes (chopped)
- 1 medium apple

Preparation:

1. Blend barley in a food processor to get flour. Transfer to a bowl and add a cup of water. Leave overnight.
2. In the morning drain excess water and then add chopped apple, raisin and chopped walnuts, prunes and apricots. Serve

Nutritional information: Dried fruit contains up to 3.5 times more fibers, vitamins, and minerals in ratio to fresh fruit.

Snack I No. 2 -Smoothie lemon and raspberries

Preparation time: 5 minutes:

Cooking time: - minutes

Number of serves: 1

Ingredients & Preparation:

1. 1 whole frozen lemon (you can cut it into small cubes and so freeze it)
2. 1 cup of raspberries
3. ½ a cup of nonfat Greek yogurt
4. 1 tablespoon of honey
5. Mix all in a blender.

Lunch No.2 - Chicken & broccoli salad

Preparation time: 10 minutes:

Cooking time: 10 minutes

Number of serves: 1

Ingredients:

- 1 breast of chicken, grilled and sliced or use any leftover chicken you might have from a roast
- ⅓ a head of broccoli
- 2 stalk, medium 7-1/2" - 8" long of celery
- 2 spring onions or scallions
- 1 green apple, preferably Granny Smith's
- 1 tsp. of mixed fresh thyme and rosemary, well chopped
- 1 tbsp of freshly squeezed lemon juice
- 1 tsp. of olive oil

Preparation:

1. In a large bowl add cooked, sliced chicken,
2. Break the broccoli into bite size florets and cook them in boiling salted water, cook for 3-5 minutes, and then drain them.

3. add to the bowl sliced celery, chopped the apple and finely sliced spring onions or scallions

4. Sprinkle over with fresh herbs and pour over lemon juice and olive oil. Mix well and serve.

Nutritional information: Broccoli is an excellent source of dietary fibers, vitamin K, C, and folate. Broccoli is loaded with flavonoids called kaempferol. This flavonoid is important for prevention and treatment of inflammatory diseases (arthritis, allergies, atherosclerosis, and even cancer).[22]

---

[22]Devi KP1, Malar DS, Nabavi SF, Sureda A, Xiao J, Nabavi SM, Daglia M. Kaempferol and inflammation: From chemistry to medicine. Department of Biotechnology, Science Campus, Alagappa University, Karaikudi india Pharmacol Res. 2015 Sep;99:1-10. http://www.ncbi.nlm.nih.gov/pubmed/25982933

Dinner No. 2 Fake cabbage spaghetti with caramelized onions in tomato sauce

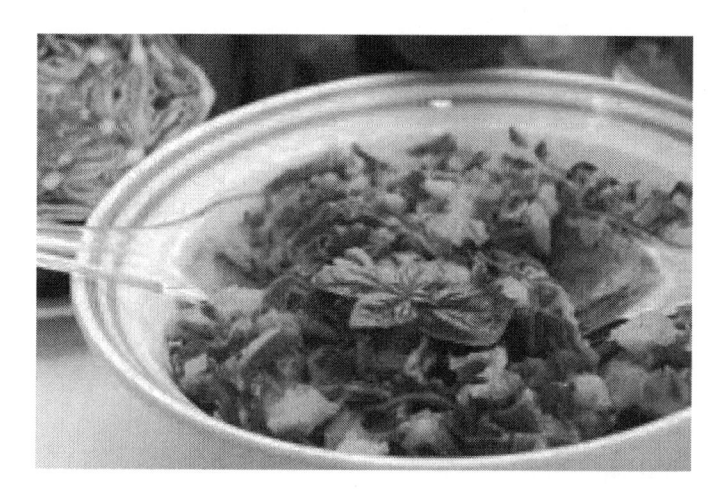

Preparation time: 10 minutes:

Cooking time: 25 minutes

Number of serves: 3

Ingredients:

- 1 head of red cabbage
- 1 small chopped onion
- 1 tsp of sugar
- 1 cup of tomato puree (homemade)
- ½ a tsp of salt
- ½ a tsp of pepper
- 1 tbsp of basil

Preparation:

1. Cut the cabbage into thin strips; blanch (in boiling water only for a few minutes).

2. Pour oil in a pan on high temperature, pour the sugar and when the sugar melts and begins to change color in brown - caramelize chopped onion (sugar caramelizing takes only 1-2 minutes).

3. Cook the onion just a little bit and immediately add cabbages "spaghetti".

4. Top up with water just enough to cover the cabbage. Cook for another 5 minutes, add the tomato paste and cook all together for another 20 minutes or until cabbage is soft. It goes great with baked potatoes.

Nutritional information: Red cabbage contains significantly more protective phytonutrients than green cabbage. Red cabbage is an excellent source of vitamin C and a very good source of manganese. Lack of manganese causes oxidant damage of cells, and can cause chronic inflammation of our body[23].

---

[23] Manganese Linus Pauling Institute Micronutrient Information Center http://lpi.oregonstate.edu/mic/minerals/manganese

Breakfast No.3 Whole meal bread with homemade spread sesame tahini

Preparation time: 10 minutes:

Cooking time: 25 minutes

Serves: 1: for each person: 2 medium slices of Italian bread, 1 oz of tahini sesame, 1 cup of green Lipton tea.

Ingredients for Tahini cream

- 3 cups of sesame seeds (1 lb.).

Preparation:

1. Preheat oven to 180°C or 350°F.

2. Place seeds in a roasting pan or rimmed cookie sheet and roast for about 10-15 minutes make sure to move them around every few minutes, so the seeds on the bottom don't burn.

3. When you have toasted your seeds, and they have cooled a bit, place them in your food processor, or a blender, and process on high until creamy, scraping down the sides as needed. It will take approx. 5-10 minutes to blend depending on your equipment.

Store your tahini in an air/tight container in the fridge. It can last up to a month. Note: To add extra creaminess use 2 or 3 tablespoons of extra virgin olive oil when blending if desired. Then you can keep it no more than 15 days in a fridge.

Nutritional information: Sesame seeds are especially high in copper, manganese, calcium, and magnesium, but the value doesn't end there; it contains sesamol, a compound that protects our DNK while it has anticancer potential, it will especially protect you from gastric cancers[24].

---

[24] Geetha T, Deol PK, Kaur IP. Role of sesamol-loaded floating beads in gastric cancers: a pharmacokinetic and biochemical evidence. Department of Pharmaceutics, UGC Centre for Advance Study, University Institute of Pharmaceutical Sciences, Panjab University, India. J Microencapsul. 2015;32(5):478-87. http://www.ncbi.nlm.nih.gov/pubmed/26268954

Snack I No.3 Blueberry and banana smoothie

Preparation time: 5 minutes:

Cooking time: - minutes

Number of serves: 1

Ingredients:

- 3 oz (80g) of frozen blueberries
- 1 medium banana
- 2 oz (56 g) of low-fat natural yogurt
- 3 fl oz (90ml) of non-fat milk
- 4 ice cubes
- Few drops of peppermint oil
- Juice from 1 freshly squeezed orange

Preparation:

1. Make sure all the ingredients are chilled before use
2. Blend fruit, yogurt, milk and juice, peppermint oil together using a hand held blender or a smoothie maker until creamy
3. Add ice cubes and blend again
4. Pour into glass and serve immediately

Lunch recipes No.3 Stuffed Sour red peppers with walnuts

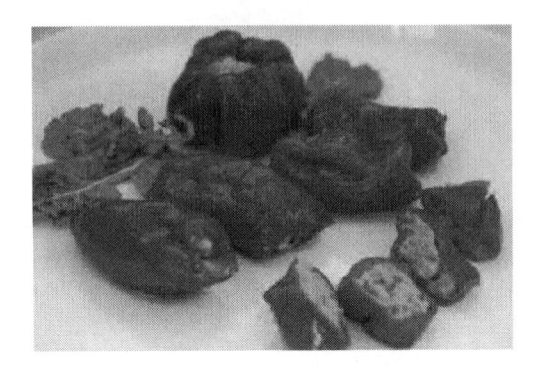

Preparation Time: 20 minutes

Baking time 25 minutes

Number of serves: 6

Ingredients:

- 12 to 15 canned or raw green or red peppers,
- 3 or 4 larger chopped onions
- 1½ a cup of chopped carrots (3-4 medium sized)
- 1 cup of coarsely ground walnuts
- 2 tbsp of chopped ginger
- ½ a cup of brown rice,
- 2 tbsp. of tomato sauce (homemade)
- 3 tbsp. of olive oil,

- Salt, pepper,

- 3 to 4 tbsp. of flour

- 1 cup of cooked and grated potatoes

Preparation:

1. Pour oil in a deeper court, about 3 tbsp, add chopped onions and carrots and fry over medium heat for about 10 minutes.

2. Add nuts. Stir and fry a little nuts release fat. Add tomato sauce, spices and fry a little bit more. Add a little water if necessary, and cook for another 5 minutes.

3. Add rice and fry it all together for a few more minutes.

4. Finally, add the grated potatoes, gently stir and remove from heat.

5. Fill the peppers with filling to ¾. Put half a teaspoon of flour in each pepper, so that the filling can't get out during cooking. You can also close it with a slice of tomato.

6. Arrange them in a baking dish, pour hot water, (peppers should be poured with just a little bit of water), cover dish with a folio, or with a lid.

7. Turn the oven to 200°C- 380°F, put the peppers in the oven and bake them for about 25 minutes. Cook over medium heat until peppers are soft.

Nutritional information: Ginger contains very potent anti-inflammatory compounds called gingerols. It plays a big role in anti-vomiting conditions and is very useful in reducing nausea and vomiting especially for pregnant women or people who have gastrointestinal disorders (gastritis, ulcer). Compound gingerols have anti-inflammatory properties, and it will relieve you from rheumatoid arthritis pain if you consume it regularly.

Dinner No.3- Mediterranean style Beef and backed potatoes

Preparation Time: 20 minutes

Baking time 35 minutes

Number of serves: 1

Ingredients:

- 4 oz (100g) of mushrooms
- 1 tbsp. of olive oil
- 1 tsp. of oregano
- 6 oz (170g) of beef steak,
- 5 onion rings,
- 1 small raw sweet red pepper,
- 1 small raw sweet green pepper,
- 1 small raw sweet yellow pepper, all sliced,
- 1 cup of chopped tomatoes,
- 1 tbsp. of olive oil,
- 1/2 cup of cooked sweet corn,
- 1 tbsp of chopped basil,
- 1 tsp of yellow mustard,

- 2 oz of white wine,

Preparation:

1. Wash mushrooms cut them in half and line them in the pan coated with olive oil and oregano and bake them for about half an hour at 200 C or 350 F.

2. Flatten out the beef steak with a meat hammer. Pour carbonated water over it and leave for half an hour in the fridge.

3. Remove the steaks from water; dry them with a napkin, after that add salt, pepper, and brush each side with mustard. Fry the steaks in a pan on the stove on medium heat to get golden brown on both sides; add a little water, a glass of white wine and cook it, covered, on low heat for about 15 min. On the end add sliced onion into it, put over steaks and cook some more.

4. When the steaks are ready, put them on a plate, cut the peppers and tomatoes into small cubes and add the corn, so they're all over the plate with the steaks. Then finally, add chopped fresh basil leaf. Serve with mushrooms baked in the oven.

Nutritional information: Peppers contain a compound named capsaicin (phytonutrient) that reduces levels of inflammation process and pain impulses from the central nervous system. Red peppers are also filled with salicylates, which are aspirin-like compounds that we usually use when we feel pain in our muscles or lower back (LBP)[25].

---

[25] Baron R, Binder A, Attal N, Casale R, Dickenson AH, Treede RD. Neuropathic low back pain in clinical practice. Division of Neurological Pain Research and Therapy, Department of

Breakfast No.4 - Polenta with yogurt

Preparation Time: 5 minutes

Cooking time 5 minutes

Number of serves: 1

Ingredients:

- 1/2 cup of organic yellow corn flour (polenta)
- a little salt and 1
- 1½ cups of water.

Preparation:

1. Put salt in boiling water, then gradually put corn flour with constant stirring on medium heat.

2. When you insert all the quantity of flour, stir until it thickens. Polenta is done when it's separated from the court in which it makes about 5 minutes to cook. Put in a plate and put yogurt over that.

Nutritional information: According to the Journal of Agricultural and Food Chemistry, food made from milled yellow corn like polenta provides a natural and excellent source of carotenoids (lipid-soluble pigments), they are a part of the antioxidant machinery and have an impact on reducing inflammation[26]. A dairy product like yogurt should be

---

Neurology, University Hospital Schleswig-Holstein, Kiel, Germany. Eur J Pain. 2016 Mar 2. doi: 10.1002/ejp.838 http://www.ncbi.nlm.nih.gov/pubmed/26935254

[26] Murillo AG, Fernandez ML. Potential of Dietary Non-Provitamin A Carotenoids in the Prevention and Treatment of Diabetic Microvascular Complications. Department of

consumed at least 11 and 14 servings per week because they are associated with decreased levels of the inflammatory marker[27].

Nutritional Sciences, University of Connecticut, Storrs, CT. <u>Adv Nutr.</u> 2016 Jan 15;7(1):14-24 http://www.ncbi.nlm.nih.gov/pubmed/26773012

[27] Panagiotakos DB, Pitsavos CH, Zampelas AD, Chrysohoou CA, Stefanadis CI. Dairy products consumption is associated with decreased levels of inflammatory markers related to cardiovascular disease in apparently healthy adults: the ATTICA study Department of Nutrition Science-Dietetics, Harokopio University, Athens, Greece <u>J Am Coll Nutr.</u> 2010 Aug;29(4):357-64. http://www.ncbi.nlm.nih.gov/pubmed/21041810

Snack I No.4 Lemon and sesame Shake

Preparation Time: 5 minutes

Cooking time - minutes

Number of serves: 1

Ingredients and Preparation:

Blend 2 teaspoons of sesame seeds that you left submerged in water overnight juice from one freshly squeezed lemon, whole grated lemon peel (organic), 1 cup yogurt, 2 tablespoons honey, 1/2 cup milk, 1/2 cup ice.

Nutritional information: Lemon decreases the acidity in your body, and it removes uric acid from your joints, which is one of the main causes of inflammation.

Lunch No.4 - Easy turkey salad

Preparation Time: 5 minutes

Cooking time - minutes

Number of serves: 1

Ingredients:

- 1 ½ a cups of mixed salad greens,
- 1 cup of chopped tomatoes,
- 3 oz of turkey breast,
- 1 cup of sliced brown mushrooms,
- 1 tsp. of dill
- 1 tbsp. of sesame oil
- 2 tbsp. of freshly squeezed lemon juice

Preparation:

Top salad greens with rest of ingredients and top with sesame oil and lemon juice dressing.

Nutritional information: Kaempferol is a flavonoid found in many edible plants including tomatoes and it's anti-oxidant/anti-inflammatory effects have been demonstrated in various disease models, including those for encephalomyelitis, diabetes, asthma, and carcinogenesis.[28]

---

[28] Rajendran P, Rengarajan T, Nandakumar N, Palaniswami R, Nishigaki Y, Nishigaki I. Kaempferol, a potential cytostatic and cure for inflammatory disorders. NPO-International Laboratory of Biochemistry, 1-166, Uchide, Nakagawa-ku, Nagoya Japan. Eur J Med Chem. 2014 Oct 30;86:103-12 http://www.ncbi.nlm.nih.gov/pubmed/25147152

Dinner No.4: Minestrone soup, Seafood with asparagus, brown rice, sour red beet salad

Preparation Time: 15 minutes

Cooking time: 35 minutes

Number of serves: 4

Ingredients for soup:

- 8 cups of water,
- 1 dice of dry chicken broth (smaller dice),
- 1 chopped onion,
- 3 cloves of chopped garlic,
- ½ a cup of sliced raw celery,
- 4 small chopped carrots,
- 2 cups of chopped kale,
- 4 oz (100g) of sliced fresh mushrooms,
- 1 large peeled tomato,
- a tbsp. of dried spices basil

Preparation:

Dissolve dry broth with water and heat in a medium soup pot; add onion in broth over medium heat for 5 minutes stirring frequently. Add garlic and continue to cook for another minute. Add rest of the ingredients except spices (basil, salt, and pepper). Bring to a boil over high heat, reduce heat to low and continue cooking, uncover for 15 minutes or until vegetables are tender. Turn off the stove and add spices. Serve.

Ingredients for Seafood with asparagus:

- a cup of chopped onion

- 3 cloves of garlic

- a cup of vegetable broth or soup

- 4 tbsp. of olive oil

- 2 tbsp. of ground ginger

- 2 cups of sliced white mushrooms,

- 8 large pieces of asparagus spear

- juice from a freshly squeezed organic lemon

- 1 chopped chili red pepper

- 1.5 lb (600g) of cod fillet, cut into strips or cubes

- 12 shrimps,

- 2 cups of sliced tomatoes

- 1 ½ a tbsp. of coriander-cilantro

Preparation:

1. Slice onion and chop garlic and let sit for 5-10 minutes to enhance its health-promoting benefits.

2. Pour oil in a deeper court, about 4 tbsp, add chopped onion and fry over medium heat for about 5 minutes.

3. Transfer sautéed onion in broth over medium high heat for next few minutes, stirring constantly.

4. Add ginger, garlic, mushrooms and asparagus. Continue to stir-fry for another 10 minutes, stirring constantly.

5. Add lemon juice, chili pepper spice, cod fillet and shrimps and stir to mix well.

6. Cover and simmer for just about 15 minutes stirring occasionally on medium heat.

7. Toss in tomatoes, cilantro, salt, and pepper. Serve with Brown Rice.

8. On the stove in a pan put 3 cups full of water, when water is boiling add ½ a cup of brown rice. Keep a lid on the pan while cooking. When it's cooked you will get a half cup of cooked rice, squeeze out all water if it remained in the cooked rice. It takes about 10 min. to cook the rice. Serve this meal with canned red beets salad.

Breakfast No.5 - Muesli with blueberries and almond milk

Preparation time- 5 minutes

Cooking time- 5 minutes

Number of serves: 1

Ingredients:

- 2 tbsp. of Organic Oat Flakes
- 1/2 cup unsweetened almond milk
- 1 tsp. ground cloves
- 2 tsp. of organic honey
- 2 tbsp. of blueberries

How to make homemade almond milk

The process essentially involves soaking almonds in water overnight or for up to two days — the longer you soak the almonds, the creamier the milk will be. Start with a ratio of 1 cup almonds to 2 cups water when making almond milk. Place the almonds in a bowl and cover with about an inch of water. They will plump as they absorb water. Let stand, uncovered, overnight or up to 2 days.

Drain the almonds from their soaking water and rinse them thoroughly under cool running water. Place the almonds in the blender and cover with 2 cups of water. Blend at the highest speed for 2 minutes. Pulse the blender a few times to break up the almonds, and then blend continuously for two minutes.

Strain the almonds. Line the strainer with either the opened nut bag or cheese cloth and place over a measuring cup. Pour the almond mixture into the strainer.

Squeeze and press with clean hands to extract as much almond milk as possible. You should get about 2 cups.

This makes milk that is roughly the consistency of 2% milk. If you'd like thinner milk, use more water next time; thicker, use less.

Preparation:

Soak oats in almond milk in the fridge overnight, at morning, stir in remaining ingredients.

Snack I No.5 Fruit shake bomb

Preparation Time: 5 minutes

Cooking time - minutes

Number of serves: 1

Ingredients:

- 1 cup of grape juice
- 2 squeezed oranges
- 2 cloves, 1 cup of apple juice
- 2 lemons – chopped
- 3 teaspoons of organic honey
- 2 pieces of cinnamon sticks

Preparation:

1. Add water, apple juice, and grape squeezed orange and squeezed lemon in a saucepan.
2. Add cloves and cinnamon. Cook juice until boiling. Remove the lid from the top, remove the cloves and cinnamon, add honey and grated lemon peel.

Nutritional information: Honey has anti-inflammatory properties and ability to calm down symptoms like a cough. Organic honey is loaded with antioxidants that can assist in the prevention of cellular damage.

Lunch No.5 Veggie broccoli and oat flakes hamburger

Preparation time: 20 minutes

Cooking time: 10 minutes

Number of serves: 3

Ingredients

- 7 oz. (200g) of oats
- 2 eggs
- 1 small chopped onion
- 3 chopped cloves of garlic
- 1 medium sized head of broccoli
- About a cup of sesame seeds
- ½ a cup of chopped celery leaf,
- 1 tbsp. of dried basil or rosemary
- ½ a tsp. of salt and pepper
- ½ a tsp. of nutmeg
- 3 tbsp. of olive oil
- About ¼ of a cup of water or less, so you can make balls.

Preparation:

1. Preheat the oven to 392°F or 200°C.

2. To soften oatmeal pour warm water over it. Take care not to add too much water; it shouldn't swim in it.

3. Add finely chopped onion and garlic.

4. Cook broccoli in salted water for about 5 minutes, drain and then mix it. If necessary, add just enough water, in which broccoli was cooked, so it's easier to blend it.

5. Add oat flakes in mashed broccoli, eggs, and spices, salt, pepper and then pour sesame seeds over it, until a mixture becomes thick enough that it can be shaped into hamburgers.

6. line up broccoli hamburger in an ovenproof dish, which you previously smeared with a little oil or baking spray and bake for about half an hour

7. Leave it for ten minutes to cool a bit and then serve as a complete lunch meal with cabbage salad and bun (included in recalculation).

Nutritional information: Sesame is one of the active compounds found in sesame-phytoestrogen or plant estrogen that can be found in the hulls of sesame seeds. Its anti-inflammatory effects have been proven in many studies in which animals were fed with sesame oil that's essential for our immune system.[29]

---

[29] Hou RC, Huang HM, Tzen JT, Jeng KC. Protective effects of sesamin and sesamolin on hypoxic neuronal and PC12 cells.Graduate Institute of Biotechnology, National Chung Hsing University, Taichung, Taiwan, Republic of China. J Neurosci Res. 2003 Oct 1;74(1):123-33. http://www.ncbi.nlm.nih.gov/pubmed/13130514

Dinner No.5 - Grilled garlic lamb chops with rosemary

Preparation time: 5 minutes

Cooking time: 15 minutes

Number of serves: 2

Ingredients:

- 4 lamb chops
- 6 tbsp. of olive oil
- 3 tbsp. of minced fresh rosemary
- 6 garlic cloves, minced
- 1 tsp. of ground black pepper

Preparation:

1. Marinate lamb in 5 tbsp. of olive oil, garlic, and rosemary for 1-4 hours.
2. Preheat oven to 400°F or 250°C.
3. Heat remaining 1 tbsp. of olive oil in a heavy large ovenproof skillet over high heat.
4. Add lamb; cook until browned, it takes about 3 minutes per side. Transfer skillet to the oven and roast lamb chops to the desired doneness, about 10 minutes for medium-rare. Transfer lamb to a platter covers and let

it rest for 5 minutes. Serve with **Spinach & Beans** as a side dish.

Ingredients for Spinach & Beans

Preparation time: 5 minutes

Cooking time: 5 minutes

Number of serves: 2

Ingredients

- 1 can of northern beans drained and rinsed
- 4 cloves of garlic
- 2 tbsp. of ground ginger
- 2 cups of fresh spinach
- 1 tbsp. of extra virgin olive oil
- 1 tsp. of tomato paste
- Pinch of salt and black cracked pepper to taste
- 1 tbsp. of fresh parsley

Preparation:

1. Heat olive oil in a skillet on low to medium heat.
2. Chop garlic and ginger into and put in skillet.
3. Rinse and drain beans and add to skillet once garlic has softened.

4. Increase heat to medium and add tomato paste, a little salt and cracked pepper. As soon as beans are heated through (few minutes), turn off heat and add spinach and fresh parsley. Serve with grilled lamb chops.

Nutritional information: Beans are full of fibers and many valuable phytonutrients and among others they have a large content of tannins (especially adzuki beans contain higher amounts of tannins). This means that beans have larger antioxidant activities, overall anti-inflammatory effects, and anti-diabetic effects than whole grains so they should be included in your meals at least twice a week.[30]

---

[30] Luo J, Cai W, Wu T1, Xu B. Phytochemical distribution in hull and cotyledon of adzuki bean (Vigna angularis L.) and mung bean (Vigna radiate L.), and their contribution to antioxidant, anti-inflammatory and anti-diabetic activities. Food Science and Technology Program, Beijing Normal University-Hong Kong Baptist University United International College, Zhuhai, Guangdong China; Food Chem. 2016 Jun 15;201:350-60 http://www.ncbi.nlm.nih.gov/pubmed/26868587

Breakfast No. 6 – Cinnamon pumpkin waffles

Preparation time: 10 minutes

Cooking time: 10 minutes

Number of serves: 5 large waffles

Ingredients:

- 1 cup pumpkin puree
- 3 eggs
- 1 tsp. of baking soda
- 1 tbsp. of cinnamon
- 2 cups of almond flour
- ¼ tsp. of salt
- 1 tsp. of anise
- 3 full tbsp. of butter

Preparation:

1. Plug in your waffle maker. Let it heat up, about 5 minutes for most waffle makers.
2. Melt butter in a saucepan a bit. Set aside 1 tbsp of it for spreading on waffle maker.

3. In a large bowl, whisk the eggs with 2 tbsp. of melted butter; add in the pumpkin puree, vanilla, cinnamon, salt and baking soda.

4. Use a rubber spatula to stir in the almond flour, until well-blended.

5. Brush the waffle maker plates with melted butter that you left aside. Place a heaping ⅓ of a cup of batter per waffle in each cavity and use a spatula to spread it. Close the lid and cook for 4-5 minutes. Repeat with all batter for waffle. Serve with more cinnamon spice.

Nutritional information: Just one tsp. of grounded cinnamon contains 46% of daily needs of mineral manganese which is considered an essential nutrient since our body requires it to function properly. Some preliminary evidence suggests that manganese can be useful in improving tendon healing. Manganese deficiency causes reduced ability of intestinal immunity, and it initiates inflammation[31].

---

[31] Jiang WD, Tang RJ, Liu Y, Kuang SY, Jiang J, Wu P, Zhao J, Zhang YA, Tang L, Tang WN, Zhou XQ, Feng L. Manganese deficiency or excess caused the depression of intestinal immunity, induction of inflammation and dysfunction of the intestinal physical barrier, as regulated by NF-κB, TOR and Nrf2 signalling, in grass carp (Ctenopharyngodon idella). Animal Nutrition Institute, Sichuan Agricultural University, Sichuan, Chengdu, China; Fish Shellfish Immunol. 2015 Oct;46(2):406-16 http://www.ncbi.nlm.nih.gov/pubmed/26072140

Snack I No. 6 – Spicy blueberry sesame smoothie

Preparation time: 10 minutes

Cooking time: - minutes

Number of serves: 1

Ingredients:

- 4 tbsp. of roasted grounded sesame seeds
- ½ a cup of water
- ½ a tsp. of grated fresh ginger
- 1 cup of frozen blueberries
- ½ a cup of kefir
- 2 tbsp. of organic honey

Preparation:

1. Place grounded sesame seeds and ½ cup of water in a blender.
2. Let soak about 15 minutes.
3. Add the blueberries, yogurt, organic honey and ginger.
4. Blend until smooth and frothy.

Nutritional information: Kefir is a natural beverage that has health-promoting bacteria and antifungal properties, therefore, kefir is very useful in the treatment of conditions such as eczema, psoriasis, and candidiasis (fungal infections), as well as some heart diseases and even AIDS, because of its ability to lift up the immune system and so fight against inflammation[32].

---

[32]Prado MR, Blandón LM, Vandenberghe LP, Rodrigues C, Castro GR, Thomaz-Soccol V, Soccol CR. Milk kefir: composition, microbial cultures, biological activities, and related products. Department of Bioprocess Engineering and Biotechnology, Federal University of Paraná Curitiba, Brazil. Front Microbiol. 2015 Oct 30;6:1177. http://www.ncbi.nlm.nih.gov/pubmed/26579086

Lunch No. 6: Halibut salad

Preparation time: 10 minutes

Cooking time: 10 minutes

Number of serves: 1

Ingredients:

- 2 cloves of chopped garlic,
- 4 outer leaf of lettuce,
- 1 fillet of halibut, fish,
- 2 fl oz of raw lemon juice,
- 1 tbsp. of dry vegetable broth,
- A bit water to dissolve broth
- 3 cups of raw Swiss chard,
- 1 tbsp. of sage spices
- 2 tbsp. of extra virgin olive oil

Preparation:

1. Press garlic and let it sit for 5 minutes to bring out its health-promoting properties.
2. Wash and dry Swiss chard and lettuce leaves. Place lettuce leaves on a plate.
3. Rub halibut with half of lemon juice.

4. Heat less than half a cup of water with veggies broth and add halibut; cover and cook for 10 minutes for each inch of thickness. Remove fish from pan and place on salad. Discard extra broth or use for soup.

5. In the same pan add chard, garlic, and sage. Put another half of lemon juice to the hot pan and heat for about 30 seconds. If you'd like to add olive oil, do so after turning off the heat. Stir mixture together for a few seconds and then drizzle over the salad.

<u>Nutritional information:</u> Swiss chard contains at least 13 different kinds of antioxidants like vitamin C and many kinds of bioflavonoid that are well-known as natural anti-inflammatory nutrients.

Dinner No.6: Risotto with shiitake mushrooms and vitamin salad

Preparation time: 10 minutes

Cooking time: 10 minutes

Number of serves: 4

Ingredients:

- 2 cups of cooked brown rice,
- 14 oz (400g) of shiitake mushrooms
- 1 large chopped red onion,
- 3 tbsp. of olive oil,
- ½ a tsp. of dried spices thyme,
- ½ a tsp. of dried rosemary

Preparation:

1. Wipe shiitake mushrooms with a clean, damp cloth to prevent sogginess.

2. Pour the oil into a preheated pan, add the chopped onion, stir and after a few min. Add chopped mushrooms. When all of "juice" evaporates from mushrooms, remove them from heat and add them to cooked rice. Mix all and add spices.

Salad Preparation: Mix all ingredients together: 2 cups of chopped white cabbage, 2 cups of red chopped cabbage, 1 cup of raw sliced red beet, 1 cup of chopped raw carrot with 4 tbsp. of extra virgin olive oil and 2 tbsp. roasted and grounded flaxseeds.

Nutritional information: Shiitake mushrooms contain strong compounds and valuable mineral named copper which is crucial to human health. These Japanese mushrooms have the natural ability to depress not only inflammation, but also all kinds of "bad" bacteria, dangerous viruses, and paradoxically, all others kinds of fungus.

Breakfast No.7: Oats muffins with berries

Preparation Time: 10 minutes.

Cooking time: 25 -35 minutes

Ingredients for 4 servings: for 12 muffins

- 3 eggs
- oz. (100g) of butter
- 7 oz. (200g) of kefir
- 1 cup of coarsely chopped almonds
- 1 cup of chopped flax seeds
- ½ a cup of oats
- 1 tsp. of baking powder
- 12 chopped prunes
- 3 tbsp of seedless raisins
- 1 cup of frozen berries (don't dissolve them previously)

Preparation:

1. Preheat the oven to 375°F or 180°C.
2. Arrange cupcake papers in a baking pan for muffins and set aside.
3. Add eggs in a mixing bowl with butter and mix it thoroughly until all ingredients are well combined.

4. Stir in mixed almonds, flax seeds, oats with baking powder, add kefir and mix until you get a smooth mixture. Add chopped prunes and frozen fruits and mix one more time.

5. Pour batter into the prepared pan but leave enough space for the growth of muffins.

6. Bake for about 20 minutes or you can check if muffins are baked by inserting a wooden pick in centers of muffins and if it comes out clean, they are baked. Cool in a pan on a wire rack for 5 minutes before removing from pan to the rack.

Nutritional information: Nuts and seeds contain high amounts of alpha-linolenic acid, which is a type of omega-3 fat. All nuts are packed with antioxidants, which can help your body fight against any inflammatory process. They are involved in repairing of the damaged cells caused by inflammation.

Snack I No.7: Ginger banana smoothie

Preparation Time: 5 minutes.

Cooking time: - minutes

Number of serves: 1

Ingredients:

- 1 sliced pineapple fruit [handwritten: BANANA?]
- 1 cup of low-fat yogurt
- 1 tbsp. of organic honey
- ½ tsp. freshly grated ginger

Blend all until smooth.

Nutritional information: Pineapples also has anti-inflammatory abilities because it contains a kind of antioxidant known as bromelain (a type of enzyme for protein-digesting). It affects on lowering of swellings, stopping redness and it has anti-tumor effects and speeds up healing time after any surgery.

Lunch No.7: White Beans baked in the oven, cabbage salad, rye bread

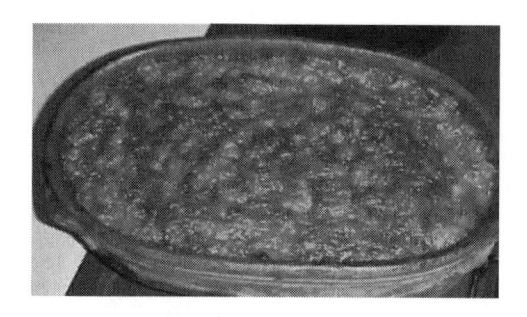

Preparation Time: 15 minutes.

Cooking time: 3 hours

Number of serves: 4

Ingredients:

- 4 cups of white beans,
- Approximately 7-8 cups of water
- 2 tbsp. of lard
- 2 large sliced or chopped onions,
- 3 cloves of chopped garlic
- 3 tbsp. of grated ginger
- 1 tsp of salt,
- 1 tsp of black pepper,
- 1 tsp of grounded red pepper

Preparation:

1. Wash and soak the beans, then leave them to stand for two hours.

2. Cook beans with 6 or 7 cups of water, and save about 2 cups of liquid in which beans were cooked (preferably water from the bottom of the container, as it contains more sludge).

3. Fry onion which is cut into thin ribs in a pan with lard on medium heat.

4. Add cooked beans and all spices, mix well.

5. If you want chili beans, add the finely chopped chili. Then move all into a deeper pan, add about 2 cups of liquid in which beans were cooked and bake on 370°F - 190°C heat for about an hour.

6. Add more water or liquid to beans during roasting if water evaporates. Bake it covered with lid or foil.

7. It goes great with cabbage salad and wholemeal bread.

Dinner No.7: Avocado & tuna salad

Preparation Time: 15 minutes.

Cooking time: 3 hours

Number of serves: 2

Ingredients:

- 6 oz of canned tuna in water
- 2 cups of avocado (1 bigger or 2 smaller)
- 1 small red onion

Dressing:

- 2 tablespoons of olive oil
- 2tbsp of squeezed lemon juice
- 2-3 tbsp. of fresh parsley
- 1 tsp. of Dill
- Pinch of Sea salt
- Pinch of black pepper

Preparation:

1. Put Tuna into a larger bowl.
2. Avocado cut in half, remove pit and cut it into small cubes, and add it to tuna. Add chopped red onion in rings due to color contrasts.

Dressing:

Add olive oil, lemon juice, pepper, salt and parsley and mix it well. Pour over prepared tuna. Serve on lettuce leaves.

Nutritional information: Seafood, especially tuna, is the only natural source of DHA and EPA; specific types of omega-3 fatty acid that improve heart health and brain function. Avocado is also fulfilled with omega 3 fatty acids, and the combination of those ingredients is one powerful weapon against inflammations.

Weekly menu plan:

S	M	T	W	T	F	S
Toasted rye bread, yogurt & scrambled egg with herbs and sesame seeds	Yoga breakfast	wholemeal bread, homemade spread sesame tahini, green tea	Polenta with yogurt	Muesli with blueberries and almond milk	Cinnamon Pumpkin waffles, green tea	Oats muffins with berries, cup of nonfat milk
Almond cupcakes	Lemon and raspberries Smoothie	Blueberry and banana smoothie	carrots and lemon smoothie	Fruit bomb Shake	Spicy blueberry sesame smoothie	Ginger pineapple smoothie
Spiced salm	Chicken &	Stuffed Sour	Easy turkey salad	veggie	Halibut	White Beans baked

	on in foil and cooked brown rice	broccoli salad	red peppers with walnuts		broccoli & oat flakes hamburger	salad	in the oven cabbage salad, rye bread
	Orange large	Apple large (Granny Smith)	2 mandarins (tangerines)	Fruit salad of 2 kiwis, 2 mandarins	1 large grapefruit	1 pomegranate	1 cup of strawberries
	Baked chickpeas, Salad with grilled zucchini	Fake cabbage spaghetti with caramelized onions in tomato sauce	Mediterranean style Beef, with grilled mushrooms	Minestrone soup, Seafood with asparagus, brown rice, sour red beet salad	Grilled garlic lamb chops with rosemary, Spinach & Beans	Risotto with shiitake mushrooms and vitamin salad	Avocado & tuna salad

Philip J. Smith

Day	Energy kcal	Protein (g)	Fats (g)	Carbohydrate (g)	Fiber (g)
Sunday	1562	93.2	70.1	143.5	19
Monday	1410	75.6	14.4	215.4	39.4
Tuesday	1907	89.3	75.5	157.9	38.3
Wednesday	2096	122.4	64.2	259.7	24.6
Thursday	1702	73.3	55.6	255.4	36.7
Friday	1799	44.8	73	214.1	26.6
Saturday	1799	100.8	49.4	242.8	41
average	1754	85.6	57.4	212.6	32.2

Note: On a 2,000-calorie-a-day diet, adults should consume between 160 to 325 grams of carbohydrates a day. Protein daily amount goes 50 to 175 grams a day based on 2000kcal intake. Fat: daily amount goes 44 to 78 grams based on 2000kcal intake.

Women need 25 grams of fiber per day, and men need 38 grams per day, according to the Institute of Medicine.

Conclusion

The best we can do for our immunity to help avoid any harmful process of inflammation is to keep it in a good shape with the aim of prevention of many diseases. We can do that with proper nutrition, regular intake of antioxidants, phytonutrient, minerals and vitamins through food. We can do this by adding spices to our regular meals. Don't forget that regular physical activity and enough sleep is also essential for proper immunity.

As I mentioned previously, spices and herbs should be used in meals to promote the natural flavor of food - not to camouflage the flavor of some specific kind of ingredients. You can use many spices and herbs in numerous kinds of dishes; however, it is essential to know what kind of herbs you can combine. When you cook without a specific recipe, always start by adding a ¼ of a teaspoon per 4 servings; Aroma cayenne pepper increases during cooking.

While it is true that most spices go well with most ingredients, there are some combinations that are particularly successful. The following list shows some of these combinations.

- ✓ Asparagus - chives, sage, tarragon, thyme.
- ✓ Beans - cumin, caraway, garlic, mint, onion, oregano, parsley, sage.
- ✓ Legumes - basil, cumin, cloves, dill, marjoram, mint, sage, thyme.

- ✓ Red meat - basil, bay leaves, coriander, cumin, curry, ginger, garlic, marjoram, onion, oregano, parsley, rosemary, sage, tarragon, thyme, mint.

- ✓ Dark green veggies - basil, dill, garlic, marjoram, oregano, tarragon, thyme.

- ✓ Cabbage - basil, cumin, chili powder paprika, cumin, dill, fennel, marjoram, sage.

- ✓ Roots (carrots, beets..) - anise, basil, chives, cinnamon, cloves, cumin, dill, marjoram, mint, parsley, sage, tarragon, thyme.

- ✓ Cauliflower - basil, cumin, shallots, cumin, dill, garlic, marjoram, parsley.

- ✓ Poultry meat - anise, basil, bay leaf, chives, cinnamon, cumin, dill, fenugreek, garlic, ginger, marjoram, onion, oregano, parsley, rosemary, saffron, sage, tarragon, thyme.

- ✓ Corn - shallots, saffron, sage, thyme.

- ✓ Eggplant - basil, cinnamon, dill, garlic, marjoram, mint, onion, oregano, parsley, sage, thyme.

- ✓ Eggs - anise, basil, cumin, cayenne red pepper, chives, coriander, dill, fennel, marjoram, oregano, parsley, rosemary, saffron, sage, tarragon, thyme.

- ✓ Fish and seafood - anise, basil, chives, dill, fennel, garlic, ginger, marjoram, oregano, parsley, rosemary, saffron, sage, tarragon, thyme.

- ✓ Fruits - anise, cinnamon, cloves, ginger, mint, rosemary.

- ✓ Rice - basil, anise, saffron, tarragon, thyme.

I hope you can see the entire picture on how to fight harmful inflammation processes. Don't forget that artificial food is full of supplements that can cause inflammation. Try to intake enough vitamins, minerals, antioxidants, dietary fibers, and everything else I mentioned, but be careful, to do this right, you need to intake it thru real, healthy food.

If you don't, you will just help inflammation attack your body and weaken your immune system, and that is the opposite of what you want to do. If you listen to what you read in this book and try to follow it, you will help your body, and improve your health, so the more you learn from this book, and the more you use what you read in it, you will be healthier, and happier.

Thank You

I hope you enjoyed the book, may I ask you for a quick favour? Leave a review here, it only takes 7 seconds:) I would really appreciate it.

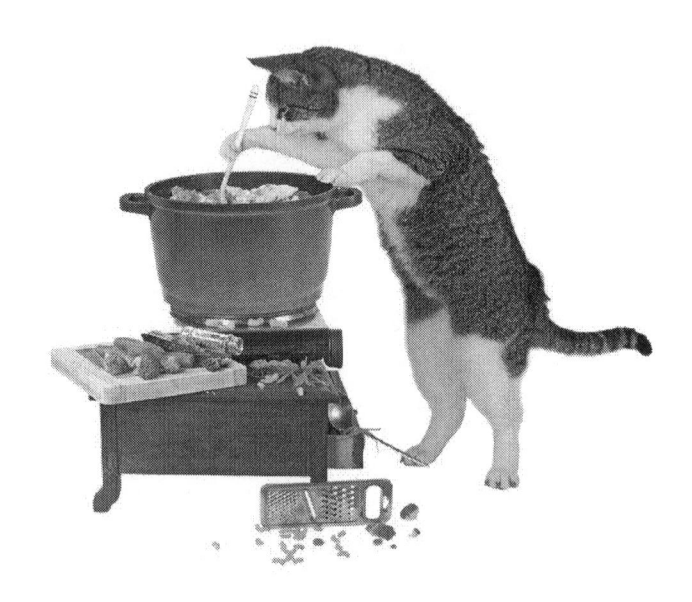

Made in the USA
Monee, IL
08 September 2024